SCARLET KLOE

Menopause Reset Guide

Ending menopause discomfort and Reviving youthfulness

Contents

Introduction

As I sit here, pen in hand, contemplating the words that will guide you through the pages of this book, my heart fills with both trepidation and excitement. For you see, I am not just a writer and researcher; I am also a woman who has traversed the intricate path of menopause. It is from the depths of my own personal journey that I write to you today, hoping to provide solace, guidance, and a glimmer of light amidst the often tumultuous storm of emotions that accompanies this transformative phase.

Menopause. The mere mention of the word evokes a myriad of emotions within me. It stirs memories of sleepless nights drenched in sweat, of tears shed for reasons I couldn't quite comprehend, and of an overwhelming sense of loss as my body bid farewell to its reproductive years. Yet, amidst the challenges and uncertainties, there was a flame within me that refused to be extinguished. It was a flame of resilience, of strength, and of an unwavering belief that this journey had the potential to unveil a renewed sense of self and an untapped wellspring of wisdom.

It is with this flame burning brightly in my heart that I invite you to embark on this poignant exploration of menopause. Together, we will traverse the peaks and valleys of this transformative phase, delving into the physical, emotional, and spiritual aspects that shape our experience. We will shed light on the often unspoken challenges, such as hot flashes that leave us feeling like we are standing in the midst of a scorching desert, or mood swings that make us question our very sanity.

But beyond the challenges lies a profound opportunity for growth and self-discovery. As women, we have endured countless transitions throughout our lives, each one leaving an indelible mark upon our souls. Menopause, with its intricate tapestry of physical and emotional changes, is no exception. It is a crossroads, a threshold, and a bridge between who we were and who we are becoming.

In sharing my personal experiences, my triumphs, and even my moments of despair, I hope to offer you a sense of camaraderie—a knowing that you are not alone on this journey. Together, we will explore strategies and insights that can ease the discomforts of menopause, revive our sense of youthfulness, and embrace the wisdom that comes with age.

My intention is not to provide a quick fix or a one-size-fits-all solution. Instead, I aim to create a space of empathy and understanding, where we can find solace in knowing that our experiences, our triumphs, and our struggles are valid and shared by countless women around the world.

As we embark on this transformative journey, let us summon the courage to face the unknown, the grace to accept the changes that unfold within us, and the strength to redefine what it means to be a vibrant, empowered, and beautiful woman in the midst of menopause.

Together, let us embrace the tears, the laughter, the uncertainties, and the joys. Let us hold hands and walk this path, shedding our old skins and stepping into the radiant light of our true selves.

With love and solidarity,

Scarlet Kloe

Understanding Menopause: A Brief Overview

Menopause, a natural biological process, marks the end of a woman's reproductive years. It is defined as the absence of menstrual periods for 12 consecutive months, indicating the depletion of ovarian follicles and the cessation of ovulation. While menopause is commonly associated with middle-aged women, it can occur anywhere between the ages of 40 and 60, with the average age being around 51.

Menopause encompasses three distinct stages: perimenopause, menopause, and postmenopause. Perimenopause is the transitional phase leading up to menopause, usually starting in a woman's 40s. During this stage, hormone levels, particularly estrogen and progesterone, fluctuate irregularly, resulting in menstrual irregularities and various physical and emotional symptoms. Menopause is officially reached when a woman has not had a menstrual period for 12 consecutive months. Postmenopause refers to the years following menopause, where hormone levels stabilize, and the body adjusts to a new hormonal balance.

Common Symptoms and Challenges

Menopause brings about a range of symptoms and challenges that can significantly impact a woman's well-being. Physical symptoms often include hot flashes, night sweats, vaginal dryness, sleep disturbances, weight gain, changes in libido, and urinary incontinence. These symptoms can vary in intensity and duration, affecting each woman differently. The hormonal fluctuations during menopause can also lead to bone loss, increasing the risk of osteoporosis.

Beyond the physical changes, menopause can also present emotional and psychological challenges. Many women experience mood swings, irritability, anxiety, and depression. The hormonal shifts, coupled with the profound transition into a new life phase, can create a sense of loss, confusion, and a reevaluation of identity and purpose. Additionally, menopause often coincides with significant life events, such as children leaving the nest or caring for aging parents, adding additional stressors to an already complex emotional landscape.

While menopause may be accompanied by physical discomforts and emotional turbulence, it is crucial to recognize it as a transformative transition rather than a period of decline. Embracing menopause involves reframing our perspective and cultivating a positive mindset about this new chapter in our lives.

Menopause can be viewed as an opportunity for self-discovery, growth, and empowerment. It is a time to celebrate the wisdom and experiences we have gained throughout our lives and to embrace the freedom that comes with no longer being governed by our reproductive cycles. By reframing menopause as a natural and necessary stage of life, we can shift our focus from the challenges to the potential for self-transformation.

Embracing menopause also involves self-care and adopting healthy lifestyle habits. Regular exercise, such as yoga or strength training, can help alleviate symptoms, improve mood, and maintain bone density. A well-balanced diet, rich in fruits, vegetables, whole grains, and lean proteins, provides the essential nutrients needed to support overall health and well-being during this transitional period. Additionally, finding stress-management techniques that work for you, such as meditation, deep breathing exercises, or engaging in hobbies, can help alleviate emotional turmoil and promote a sense of inner calm.

Support systems play a vital role in navigating the menopause journey. Sharing experiences with friends, joining support groups, or seeking guidance from healthcare professionals can provide a sense of camaraderie and reassurance. Surrounding ourselves with understanding and empathetic individuals can help us feel validated, less alone, and better equipped to face the challenges that arise during this time.

Understanding menopause is essential for women to navigate this transformative phase with knowledge, grace, and resilience. By embracing menopause as a transition, we can reframe our experiences, foster self-compassion, and focus on the potential for personal growth and empowerment. Menopause may mark the end of one phase, but it opens doors to new possibilities, wisdom, and a renewed sense of self.

Part I: Preparing for Your Menopause Reset

Welcome to Part I of "Menopause Reset Guide : Ending Menopause Discomfort and Reviving Youthfulness." In this section, we will delve into the essential aspects of preparing yourself for a successful menopause reset.

As we embark on this transformative journey together, let us prepare ourselves mentally, physically, and emotionally for the menopause reset ahead. By adopting a positive mindset and nurturing our bodies and minds, we can navigate through menopause with ease, ending discomfort and reviving our inner youthfulness. Get ready to embark on a remarkable path of self-discovery and empowerment as we delve into Part I.

Accepting the Change: Embracing a Positive Mindset

As I embarked on my own journey through menopause, one of the most crucial steps I took was to accept the change and embrace a positive mindset. Menopause can be a time of uncertainty and physical and emotional fluctuations, but by shifting my perspective and cultivating a positive outlook, I found the strength and resilience to navigate this transformative phase with grace and optimism.

Accepting the change begins with acknowledging that menopause is a natural and inevitable part of a woman's life. It is a transition that signifies the end of our reproductive years and marks a new chapter filled with possibilities. Initially, I struggled with the idea of letting go of my fertility and the societal expectations that came with it. However, I soon realized that menopause is not a sign of weakness or decline but a testament to the wisdom and experience we have gained throughout our lives.

Embracing a positive mindset means reframing menopause as a time of empowerment and self-discovery. Rather than dwelling on the physical symptoms and limitations, I chose to focus on the opportunities for personal growth and renewal that menopause presents. This shift in mindset allowed me to celebrate the changes happening within my body and embrace the uniqueness of my journey.

It is essential to remember that embracing a positive mindset does not mean denying or dismissing the challenges that come with menopause. Instead, it is about finding the silver linings, seeking support, and proactively managing the symptoms. I found solace in connecting with other women who were also going through menopause, sharing our experiences, and providing each other with understanding and encouragement. Together, we created a network of support that empowered us to face the challenges head-on.

In my personal experience, cultivating a positive mindset involved practicing self-compassion and self-care. I allowed myself to acknowledge and honor the emotions that surfaced during this transition, whether it was frustration, sadness, or even moments of joy. Journaling, meditation, and engaging in creative outlets such as writing and painting became therapeutic practices that helped me process my thoughts and emotions.

Additionally, I discovered the power of self-care in nurturing my overall well-being. Prioritizing activities that brought me joy, such as spending time in nature, practicing yoga, or indulging in a favorite hobby, allowed me to reconnect with myself and find balance amidst the changes. By caring for my physical, emotional, and spiritual needs, I fostered a positive mindset that permeated every aspect of my menopause journey.

Embracing a positive mindset during menopause is a journey in itself, filled with ups and downs. It requires patience, self-reflection, and a willingness to embrace change. As I opened myself up to new possibilities and embraced the transformation happening within me, I discovered a renewed sense of purpose and a deeper appreciation for the resilience of the female body.

Accepting the change and embracing a positive mindset are pivotal steps in preparing for your menopause reset. By shifting your perspective, celebrating the wisdom gained throughout your life, and practicing self-compassion and self-care, you can navigate the challenges of menopause with grace and optimism. Embracing this transformative phase allows you to discover new strengths, explore new passions, and embark on a journey of self-discovery and renewed vitality.

Shifting Perspectives: Menopause as a Natural Process

When I first embarked on my journey through menopause, I must admit that I had some preconceived notions and fears about this phase of life. Like many women, I had absorbed societal messages that portrayed menopause as something to dread—a time of decline, discomfort, and loss. However, as I delved deeper into my own experience and conducted research, I discovered a different perspective—one that allowed me to see menopause as a natural process of transformation and growth.

Menopause, at its core, is a biological milestone that marks the end of our reproductive years. It is a natural transition that every woman goes through, signaling a shift in hormonal balance and the cessation of menstruation. Instead of viewing it as an abrupt halt or a disruption to our lives, I began to see it as a gradual and necessary progression. Menopause represents a new chapter, offering opportunities for self-reflection, self-care, and embracing the wisdom that comes with age.

Embracing menopause as a natural process starts with reframing our thoughts and beliefs about aging. Society often places immense pressure on women to maintain a youthful appearance and conform to narrowly defined standards of beauty. However, as I navigated my own menopause journey, I realized the importance of celebrating the changes that occur within our bodies. Each wrinkle, gray hair, and shift in our physical appearance tells a story—a testament to a life lived, challenges overcome, and wisdom gained. Embracing these changes allows us to embrace our authentic selves and reject the unrealistic expectations imposed upon us.

In addition to shifting our perspective on aging, it is crucial to recognize that menopause is a normal part of the female life cycle. It is not a flaw or a medical condition that needs to be fixed but rather a natural occurrence that deserves acceptance and understanding. By viewing menopause through this lens, we can approach it with a sense of curiosity, openness, and even gratitude for the opportunities it presents.

For me, shifting my perspective meant letting go of the fear and uncertainty that initially accompanied the onset of menopause. I began to view it as a time to prioritize my well-being and invest in self-care practices that would support me through this transition. I sought out information, connected with other women who were going through similar experiences, and learned from their stories. Sharing our experiences and supporting one another creates a sense of community, reassurance, and empowerment as we navigate this transformative phase together.

In conclusion, shifting our perspective on menopause as a natural process allows us to embrace the changes with acceptance, gratitude, and a sense of empowerment. It is a time to let go of societal expectations, celebrate our unique journey, and prioritize self-care. By embracing menopause as a natural part of life, we can unlock the potential for personal growth, self-discovery, and the revival of our inner youthfulness.

Overcoming Stereotypes and Societal Expectations

As women approaching menopause, we often find ourselves confronted with a myriad of stereotypes and societal expectations that can influence how we perceive and experience this transformative phase of life. Overcoming these stereotypes and challenging societal norms is an essential step in preparing ourselves for a menopause reset that embraces our individuality, strength, and resilience. Drawing from my personal experiences, I have learned the importance of breaking free from these constraints and defining my own narrative.

One prevalent stereotype surrounding menopause is the notion that it signifies the end of our attractiveness or desirability. Society often perpetuates the belief that menopausal women are no longer youthful, vibrant, or relevant. This can lead to feelings of self-doubt and a loss of self-esteem. However, it is crucial to recognize that beauty and vitality are not determined solely by age or reproductive capabilities. By challenging these stereotypes, we can redefine beauty on our own terms and celebrate the wisdom, experience, and confidence that come with age.

I vividly remember a time when I struggled with these societal expectations. I felt a sense of pressure to maintain a youthful appearance and conform to societal standards of beauty. However, as I embarked on my menopause journey, I realized that true beauty emanates from within and is not confined by external appearances. Embracing my changing body and allowing myself to let go of societal expectations was liberating. I discovered that my value as a woman extends far beyond my physical appearance and that my self-worth is not tied to societal norms.

Another stereotype that women often face during menopause is the assumption that this phase of life signifies a decline in productivity or capability. It is not uncommon to encounter ageism in various spheres, such as the workplace or personal relationships. However, it is crucial to challenge these biases and recognize the wealth of experience, knowledge, and skills that we bring to the table. Menopause can be a time of increased self-awareness, clarity of purpose, and renewed focus, allowing us to excel in new and unexpected ways.

I recall a professional setting where I encountered age-related bias during my menopause transition. Instead of succumbing to these assumptions, I seized the opportunity to showcase my expertise and adaptability. By challenging preconceived notions and demonstrating my value through my contributions, I shattered the stereotype that menopause equates to diminished capabilities. It was a powerful reminder that menopause does not mark the end of our professional or personal growth but rather a new chapter filled with potential and opportunity.

Overcoming stereotypes and societal expectations requires a conscious effort to rewrite the narrative surrounding menopause. By embracing our uniqueness, celebrating our accomplishments, and challenging the status quo, we pave the way for a more inclusive and empowering experience of menopause. It is through our individual stories and collective voices that we can inspire and support other women in embracing their own menopause journeys.

In conclusion, preparing for your menopause reset involves overcoming stereotypes and societal expectations that can hinder our personal growth and well-being. By rejecting the notion that menopause diminishes our worth or capabilities, we can redefine our own narratives and embrace this transformative phase with confidence and empowerment. Let us break free from the constraints imposed by society, celebrate our wisdom and experience, and pave the way for a menopause journey that honors our individuality and resilience.

Cultivating Self-Compassion and Self-Care

As we prepare for our menopause reset, it is essential to cultivate a mindset of self-compassion and prioritize self-care. Menopause brings about significant changes, both physically and emotionally, and navigating this transition requires us to be kind and gentle with ourselves. Drawing from my personal experiences, I have learned that self-compassion and self-care are powerful tools that can help us embrace this phase of life with grace and resilience.

Menopause can sometimes feel like a roller coaster ride, with its share of ups and downs. It is during these challenging moments that self-compassion becomes crucial. Rather than judging ourselves for the symptoms we experience or comparing ourselves to others, it is important to offer ourselves kindness and understanding. Recognizing that menopause is a natural and inevitable part of our journey allows us to approach it with acceptance and self-love.

One way to cultivate self-compassion is by acknowledging and validating our emotions. Menopause can bring about a whirlwind of feelings, including sadness, frustration, and even a sense of loss. It is vital to create a safe space where we can freely express these emotions without judgment. Whether through journaling, talking to a trusted friend or therapist, or engaging in creative outlets such as art or music, giving ourselves permission to feel and process our emotions can be incredibly healing.

Self-care is another integral aspect of preparing for our menopause reset. As women, we often prioritize the needs of others above our own, but during this transformative period, it is crucial to make self-care a priority. Taking the time to nurture our physical, emotional, and spiritual well-being can have a profound impact on how we navigate menopause.

Physically, self-care may involve adopting a nourishing diet and engaging in regular exercise. Menopause can bring about changes in our metabolism and body composition, and by fueling our bodies with nutritious foods and engaging in physical activities we enjoy, we can support our overall well-being. Incorporating practices such as yoga or tai chi can also help us stay flexible and reduce stress levels.

Emotional self-care is equally important. During menopause, we may find ourselves grappling with mood swings, irritability, or feelings of anxiety. Engaging in activities that bring us joy and provide emotional nourishment can be transformative. This could include reading a favorite book, practicing mindfulness or meditation, spending time in nature, or pursuing hobbies and passions that bring us a sense of fulfillment.

Additionally, nurturing our spiritual well-being can provide a sense of grounding and inner peace during the menopause transition. This may involve exploring practices such as meditation, prayer, or connecting with a supportive community that shares our values and beliefs. Taking time for introspection and reflection can help us gain a deeper understanding of ourselves and find meaning in this transformative phase of life.

In my personal journey, cultivating self-compassion and self-care has been a lifeline during menopause. By approaching myself with kindness, embracing my emotions, and making self-care a priority, I have found the strength and resilience to navigate the challenges that come with this transition. It is through self-compassion and self-care that we can lay the foundation for our menopause reset, allowing us to embrace this transformative journey with grace, confidence, and a renewed sense of self.

Remember, as you prepare for your menopause reset, be gentle with yourself, prioritize self-care, and embrace the transformative power of self-compassion. You deserve to navigate this transition with love and kindness, and by doing so, you will unlock the potential for renewed vitality and embrace the beauty of this next chapter in your life.

Nurturing Your Body

In this section, we will explore the crucial aspect of nurturing your body during the menopause journey. By adopting a holistic approach, we can balance hormones, enhance our physical well-being, and alleviate the discomfort often associated with menopause.

One of the fundamental pillars of nurturing your body during menopause is through nutrition. The foods we consume play a vital role in balancing hormones and managing menopause symptoms. We will explore dietary recommendations that focus on incorporating nutrient-rich foods, balancing macronutrients, and incorporating specific superfoods that can alleviate symptoms such as hot flashes, mood swings, and fatigue.

Our body undergoes significant hormonal changes. The ovaries gradually produce fewer hormones, particularly estrogen and progesterone, leading to the cessation of menstrual cycles. This transition can bring about various physical and emotional symptoms, including hot flashes, night sweats, mood swings, sleep disturbances, vaginal dryness, and decreased libido.

It's crucial to recognize that menopause is a natural aspect of the aging process and does not necessitate medical treatment. Nevertheless, many women experience bothersome symptoms during this time, and there are options available to alleviate them. Moreover, by nourishing our bodies internally, we can provide the necessary foundation for optimal well-being throughout this transformative phase.

Balancing Hormones Naturally

As I experienced my own menopause journey, I became acutely aware of the impact these hormonal fluctuations can have on our overall well-being. Fortunately, there are various natural approaches we can adopt to help balance our hormones and alleviate the discomfort associated with menopause.

One key aspect of balancing hormones naturally is paying attention to our diet. Incorporating foods that support hormonal balance and knowing when to eat can make a significant difference in managing menopause symptoms.

However, through my own journey, I've learned that adjusting my eating patterns can have a profound impact on managing these symptoms.

Intermittent fasting, a practice that involves cycling between periods of eating and fasting, has emerged as a potential game-changer for menopausal women. By extending the overnight fasting period and compressing the eating window, our bodies are given the opportunity to reset and rejuvenate.

Personally, I found that adopting a 16:8 fasting protocol, where I fast for 16 hours and consume all my meals within an 8-hour window, worked wonders. Not only did it help me shed a few stubborn pounds that seemed to cling on during menopause, but it also brought about a sense of mental clarity and increased energy.

Allowing my body an extended break from digestion overnight seemed to recalibrate my hormone levels, leading to fewer hot flashes and improved sleep quality. It's as if my body found a newfound balance, helping me navigate this transitional phase with greater ease.

But it's not just about when we eat; it's also about what we eat. Incorporating a wholesome, nutrient-dense diet during the eating window can further enhance the benefits. Including plenty of fruits, vegetables, whole grains, lean proteins, and healthy fats can provide the necessary nourishment and support our bodies need during menopause.

Personally, I found that increasing my intake of foods rich in phytoestrogens, such as soy, flaxseeds, and legumes, helped to regulate my hormone levels and reduce hot flashes and night sweats. Additionally, consuming a variety of fruits, vegetables, and whole grains provided me with essential nutrients and antioxidants, supporting overall hormonal health.

Regular exercise is another powerful tool for naturally balancing hormones during menopause. Engaging in physical activity helps to regulate hormone levels, reduce stress, and maintain a healthy weight. From my personal experience, I found that incorporating activities like yoga, brisk walking, and strength training into my routine not only improved my physical well-being but also had a positive impact on my mood and energy levels.

In addition to dietary and exercise considerations, exploring alternative therapies and complementary medicine can provide further support in balancing hormones naturally. For instance, herbal supplements like black cohosh and red clover have been shown to help manage menopause symptoms by mimicking the effects of estrogen in the body. However, it is important to consult with a healthcare professional before incorporating any supplements into your routine, as they may interact with other medications or have individual contraindications.

Moreover, mind-body practices such as meditation, deep breathing exercises, and mindfulness can significantly contribute to hormonal balance. These practices help reduce stress levels, improve sleep quality, and enhance overall well-being. Taking time for myself to engage in these activities allowed me to connect with my inner self, reduce anxiety, and create a sense of calm amidst the hormonal changes.

While it is essential to embrace natural approaches to balance hormones during menopause, it is equally important to remember that every woman's experience is unique. What worked for me may not work for everyone. It is crucial to listen to your body and find the strategies that resonate with you personally. Consulting with a healthcare provider who specializes in menopause management can provide valuable guidance and ensure that the approach you choose aligns with your specific needs.

As you embark on your journey to balance hormones naturally, remember that it is a process of self-discovery and experimentation. Be patient with yourself, and allow time to understand what works best for your body. By adopting a holistic approach that encompasses nutrition, exercise, alternative therapies, and self-care practices, you can support your body in achieving hormonal balance and pave the way for a smoother menopause experience.

Nutrition and Menopause: Foods to Embrace and Avoid

As we navigate through menopause, nurturing our bodies becomes of utmost importance. Our diet plays a significant role in supporting our overall well-being and managing the symptoms that accompany this transformative phase. As a woman who has experienced menopause and explored various dietary choices, I have come to appreciate the impact that nutrition can have on alleviating discomfort and reviving youthfulness.

During menopause, hormonal fluctuations can lead to a range of symptoms such as hot flashes, mood swings, and weight gain. By adopting a holistic approach to nutrition, we can optimize our hormonal balance, support our energy levels, and promote overall health. Let's delve into the foods we should embrace and those we should avoid to nurture our bodies during menopause.

Embracing Nutrient-Dense Foods:

1. Phytoestrogen-rich Foods: Phytoestrogens are plant-based compounds that mimic estrogen in the body. They can help balance hormone levels and reduce menopause symptoms. Incorporate foods such as soy products, flaxseeds, chickpeas, lentils, and whole grains into your diet.

- Personal Experience: I found that including soy milk and tofu in my meals helped alleviate hot flashes and improve my overall well-being.

1. Calcium-Rich Foods: Menopause can increase the risk of bone loss and osteoporosis. Consuming adequate calcium is crucial for maintaining strong bones. Include dairy products, leafy greens, almonds, sesame

seeds, and fortified plant-based milks in your diet.

- Personal Experience: Adding more leafy greens like kale and broccoli to my meals and incorporating almond milk into my daily routine helped support my bone health.

1. Omega-3 Fatty Acids: These healthy fats have anti-inflammatory properties and can support heart health and brain function. Include fatty fish like salmon and sardines, walnuts, chia seeds, and flaxseeds in your diet.

- Personal Experience: Incorporating walnuts and flaxseeds into my snacks and meals not only improved my brain function but also helped alleviate joint pain and inflammation.

1. Colorful Fruits and Vegetables: Aim for a variety of colorful fruits and vegetables to ensure a wide range of vitamins, minerals, and antioxidants. These nutrients can support immune function and provide essential nourishment for your body.

- Personal Experience: I discovered the benefits of incorporating berries, citrus fruits, leafy greens, and vibrant vegetables like bell peppers and carrots into my meals. They not only provided a burst of flavor but also enhanced my overall vitality.

Avoiding Trigger Foods:

1. Processed and Sugary Foods: Processed foods and those high in added sugars can lead to inflammation, weight gain, and mood swings. Limit your intake of packaged snacks, sugary drinks, refined grains, and desserts.

- Personal Experience: I noticed that reducing my consumption of sugary treats and processed snacks helped stabilize my energy levels and improved my overall mood.

1. Caffeine and Alcohol: Both caffeine and alcohol can disrupt sleep patterns, exacerbate hot flashes, and contribute to dehydration. Limit your intake of coffee, tea, energy drinks, and alcoholic beverages.

- Personal Experience: I found that reducing my caffeine intake and limiting alcohol consumption in the evening greatly improved the quality of my sleep and reduced night sweats.

1. Spicy Foods: Spicy foods can trigger hot flashes and worsen existing symptoms. Consider reducing your consumption of spicy peppers, chili, and hot sauces.

- Personal Experience: I noticed a significant decrease in the frequency and intensity of hot flashes when I minimized my consumption of spicy foods.

Remember, each woman's experience with menopause is unique, so it's essential to listen to your body and adjust your diet accordingly. Consulting with a healthcare professional or a registered dietitian can provide personalized guidance based on your specific needs.

By embracing nutrient-dense foods and avoiding triggers, we can nurture our bodies during menopause and optimize our overall well-being. As you embark on your menopause reset, explore new recipes, and experiment with different foods to find what works best for you. Nourish yourself from within and savor the journey of revitalizing your body and embracing your inner youthfulness.

The Importance of Exercise and Physical Activity

When it comes to navigating menopause and revitalizing your body, exercise and physical activity play a vital role. As a woman who has personally experienced the transformative power of exercise during menopause, I can attest to its positive impact on both physical and emotional well-being. Incorporating regular exercise into your routine can help alleviate menopause symptoms, improve overall health, and revive your sense of youthfulness.

During menopause, our bodies undergo hormonal changes that can contribute to weight gain, decreased bone density, and loss of muscle tone. Engaging in exercise not only helps manage weight but also strengthens bones, muscles, and joints. I vividly recall my own journey of discovering the importance of exercise during menopause. By incorporating a combination of cardiovascular activities, strength training, and flexibility exercises, I experienced increased energy levels, improved sleep quality, and enhanced overall physical fitness.

Cardiovascular exercises, such as brisk walking, jogging, swimming, or cycling, have numerous benefits for women going through menopause. These activities increase heart rate, improve circulation, and promote the release of endorphins, which can alleviate mood swings and boost overall mental well-being. Engaging in cardiovascular exercise not only helps manage weight but also reduces the risk of cardiovascular diseases that can become more prevalent during menopause.

Strength training exercises are equally important during this stage of life. By incorporating resistance exercises, such as lifting weights or using resistance bands, you can help maintain muscle mass, increase bone density, and improve overall strength. I found that strength training exercises not only enhanced my physical capabilities but also instilled a sense of empowerment and confidence as I witnessed my body becoming stronger and more resilient.

Flexibility exercises, such as yoga or Pilates, can help alleviate muscle tension, improve posture, and enhance joint mobility. As I engaged in these activities, I noticed a significant reduction in the joint stiffness and muscle tightness that often accompany menopause. Flexibility exercises also provided a space for mindfulness and self-reflection, allowing me to find moments of tranquility and balance amidst the changes I was experiencing.

It's important to find activities that you enjoy and that fit your lifestyle. Whether it's dancing, hiking, gardening, or participating in group fitness classes, incorporating exercise into your daily routine should be a joyful and fulfilling experience. Find activities that bring you joy and make you feel connected to your body.

When starting an exercise routine during menopause, it's important to listen to your body and gradually increase intensity and duration. Consulting with a healthcare professional or a certified fitness trainer can help you develop a personalized exercise plan that suits your needs and takes into account any specific health considerations.

Incorporating exercise into your menopause journey is not just about physical health; it also has a profound impact on emotional well-being. Exercise releases endorphins, which can elevate mood, reduce anxiety and stress, and improve overall mental well-being. Personally, I found that engaging in regular exercise helped me better manage the emotional ups and downs often associated with menopause, providing a sense of balance and inner peace.

In conclusion, exercise and physical activity are essential components of a holistic approach to menopause. By incorporating cardiovascular exercises, strength training, and flexibility exercises into your routine, you can manage weight, improve bone density and muscle tone, and enhance overall well-being. Remember to find activities that you enjoy and listen to your body's needs as you embark on this empowering journey. Through exercise, you can revitalize your body, navigate menopause with grace, and revive your sense of youthfulness and vitality.

Exploring Alternative Therapies and Complementary Medicine

Menopause brings about hormonal fluctuations and physical changes that can sometimes be challenging to manage. While traditional medical approaches can provide valuable solutions, exploring alternative therapies and complementary medicine can offer additional support and relief. In this section, we will dive into the realm of alternative therapies and discuss my personal experiences with these approaches during my own menopause journey.

1. Acupuncture: Acupuncture is an ancient Chinese practice that involves the insertion of thin needles into specific points of the body. It is believed to restore the balance of energy flow, known as Qi. During my menopause journey, I decided to give acupuncture a try after hearing positive experiences from friends. I found that regular acupuncture sessions helped alleviate hot flashes and improve my overall sense of well-being. The soothing nature of the treatment provided a sense of calm during a time of hormonal fluctuations.

2. Herbal Medicine: Herbal remedies have been used for centuries to address various health concerns, including menopause symptoms. Personally, I explored the use of herbal supplements such as black cohosh, red clover, and evening primrose oil. While individual results may vary, incorporating these herbs into my routine seemed to reduce the frequency and intensity of hot flashes. It is important to consult with a qualified herbalist or healthcare professional before starting any herbal remedies to ensure they are suitable for your specific needs.

3. Mind-Body Practices: Mind-body practices such as yoga, meditation, and deep breathing exercises have proven to be effective in managing stress, promoting relaxation, and enhancing overall well-being. During my menopause journey, I incorporated regular yoga and meditation sessions into my routine. Not only did these practices help me find moments of calm amidst the hormonal storm, but they also improved my flexibility and mental clarity. Mind-body practices can be a valuable tool in navigating the emotional and physical changes that come with

menopause.

4. Traditional Chinese Medicine (TCM): TCM is a comprehensive system of healing that encompasses acupuncture, herbal medicine, dietary recommendations, and lifestyle adjustments. Drawing from ancient Chinese wisdom, TCM aims to restore balance and harmony within the body. I consulted with a TCM practitioner who tailored a treatment plan specifically for my menopause symptoms. Through a combination of acupuncture, herbal remedies, and dietary adjustments, I experienced a noticeable reduction in hot flashes and improved overall energy levels.

5. Massage Therapy: Massage therapy can be a soothing and therapeutic way to alleviate muscle tension, improve circulation, and promote relaxation during menopause. Regular massages helped me relieve physical discomfort, reduce stress levels, and improve my sleep quality. Whether it was a full-body massage or focusing on specific areas like the neck and shoulders, the power of touch played a significant role in my menopause journey.

It is important to note that while alternative therapies and complementary medicine can offer relief and support during menopause, it is essential to consult with qualified practitioners and healthcare professionals. They can guide you in selecting the most appropriate therapies for your specific needs and ensure that they complement any other treatments or medications you may be using.

Remember, everyone's experience with alternative therapies may vary, and what works for one person may not work for another. It is a journey of exploration and self-discovery, so be open to trying different approaches and finding what resonates with you. By nurturing your body through a holistic approach that includes alternative therapies, you can find additional support and relief during your menopause journey.

Part II: Strategies for Ending Menopause Discomfort

Welcome to Part II of "Menopause Reset Guide : Ending Menopause Discomfort and Reviving Youthfulness." In this section, we will delve into effective strategies and techniques to alleviate the discomfort that often accompanies the menopause journey. By understanding and managing the common symptoms of menopause, we can enhance our overall well-being and regain a sense of comfort and vitality.

Taming the Hormone Roller Coaster: Managing Symptoms

Entering the menopause phase brings with it a roller coaster ride of hormonal changes that can manifest in various physical and emotional symptoms. As someone who has experienced this firsthand, I understand the challenges that accompany these hormonal fluctuations. In this section, we will explore effective strategies for managing the symptoms and regaining a sense of balance and well-being.

One of the most common and disruptive symptoms experienced during menopause is **hot flashes** and **night sweats**. These sudden waves of intense heat can be accompanied by profuse sweating, rapid heartbeat, and feelings of anxiety. To manage these episodes, it can be helpful to identify triggers such as spicy foods, caffeine, or stress, and make necessary lifestyle adjustments.

Personally, I found that practicing deep breathing exercises and mindfulness techniques helped me remain calm and reduce the intensity and frequency of hot flashes.

It is also important to maintain a cool and comfortable environment. Keep your bedroom well-ventilated, invest in breathable bedding, and consider using a fan or air conditioner to regulate the temperature. Dress in layers, so you can easily remove or add clothing as needed.

Avoid triggers that can exacerbate hot flashes, such as spicy foods, caffeine, and alcohol. Instead, focus on incorporating cooling foods like cucumbers, watermelon, and mint into your diet. Stay hydrated throughout the day, as dehydration can intensify hot flashes.

Regular exercise has been a game-changer for me. Engaging in physical activity not only helps regulate body temperature but also improves overall well-being. Incorporate aerobic exercises, like brisk walking or swimming, into your routine, and explore mind-body practices such as yoga or tai chi for their calming effects.

Stress Management also plays a crucial role. Stress can trigger or worsen hot flashes and night sweats. Explore relaxation techniques such as deep breathing exercises, meditation, or gentle stretching to help calm your mind and body. Prioritize self-care activities that bring you joy and help you unwind.

Handling Sleep Disturbances

Sleep disturbances and insomnia can also plague menopausal women, leaving them feeling tired and fatigued. Hormonal imbalances, night sweats, and anxiety can contribute to difficulty falling asleep or staying asleep throughout the night. Establishing a consistent bedtime routine and creating a sleep-friendly environment can help promote better sleep. Personally, I found that incorporating relaxation techniques such as a warm bath, reading a book, or practicing gentle yoga before bed helped me unwind and improve my sleep quality.

Vaginal dryness and changes in sexual function are also common concerns during menopause. These changes can impact self-esteem, intimate relationships, and overall quality of life. Open and honest communication with your partner about these changes is essential. Additionally, using lubricants, moisturizers, and seeking guidance from healthcare professionals can help address and manage these symptoms effectively.

Mood Swings and Emotional Well-being

Menopause is often accompanied by mood swings and emotional fluctuations that can feel overwhelming and disruptive. As a woman who has experienced these challenges firsthand, I understand the impact they can have on our overall well-being. However, it is important to remember that there are strategies and approaches that can help us effectively manage and overcome these mood swings, allowing us to maintain emotional well-being during this transformative phase.

Mood swings during menopause can range from mild irritability and moodiness to more severe bouts of anxiety or depression. The hormonal changes that occur during menopause can disrupt the delicate balance of neurotransmitters in the brain, leading to these emotional fluctuations. However, it is essential to recognize that mood swings are not a reflection of personal weakness or failure but rather a natural response to the changes happening within our bodies.

One strategy for managing mood swings is to prioritize self-care and make time for activities that promote emotional well-being. Engaging in activities that bring you joy, such as hobbies, creative pursuits, or spending time in nature, can help lift your spirits and provide a sense of fulfillment. It is also beneficial to establish a consistent self-care routine that includes practices such as meditation, deep breathing exercises, or journaling to help calm the mind and cultivate inner peace.

Another valuable approach is seeking support from loved ones or joining a support group specifically for menopausal women. Sharing your experiences with others who are going through similar challenges can provide a sense of validation, understanding, and camaraderie. It can be empowering to know that you are not alone in navigating the emotional ups and downs of menopause. Additionally, confiding in a trusted friend or family member can offer a safe space for expressing your emotions and seeking guidance.

In my personal journey, I found that incorporating stress management techniques was instrumental in managing mood swings. Chronic stress can exacerbate menopause symptoms and intensify emotional fluctuations. Exploring stress reduction techniques such as mindfulness, yoga, or regular exercise can help promote a sense of calm and improve overall emotional well-being. Taking the time to prioritize self-reflection, identify stress triggers, and implement healthy coping mechanisms can be transformative in maintaining a stable emotional state.

For some women, seeking professional help, such as therapy or counseling, may be beneficial in managing mood swings and emotional challenges during menopause. A therapist can provide a safe and supportive environment for exploring and processing emotions, offering guidance and strategies to navigate this transitional phase. They can also help identify any underlying issues that may be contributing to mood swings and provide tailored solutions to promote emotional well-being.

It is important to remember that managing mood swings during menopause is an ongoing process. What works for one person may not work for another, so it is essential to be patient and open to trying different strategies. Embracing self-compassion and self-acceptance throughout this journey is paramount. Menopause is a time of transition, growth, and self-discovery, and by actively addressing our emotional well-being, we can emerge stronger, more resilient, and with a renewed sense of inner balance.

Experiencing mood swings during menopause is a common and understandable phenomenon. By prioritizing self-care, seeking support, managing stress, and exploring professional guidance, we can effectively navigate the emotional challenges of this phase.

By implementing these strategies and exploring other options such as herbal remedies, mindfulness practices, or hormone replacement therapy, you can find relief from menopause discomfort and regain a sense of control over your well-being. While it may take time to find the right combination of approaches, with persistence and self-care, you can effectively manage the symptoms of the hormone roller coaster and experience a more comfortable menopause journey.

Remember, managing menopause symptoms is not a one-size-fits-all approach. Each woman's experience is unique, and it may require some trial and error to find the strategies that work best for you. It is essential to listen to your body, be patient with yourself, and seek professional guidance if needed. Remember, you are not alone in this journey, and there is support available to help you navigate through these challenges.

In the next section, we will explore strategies for protecting your skeletal health and addressing the concerns of bone loss commonly associated with menopause. So let's continue our journey together, armed with knowledge and the determination to overcome menopause discomfort and embrace a revitalized sense of youthfulness.

The Battle Against Bone Loss: Protecting Your Skeletal Health

In this section, we will delve into the critical topic of protecting your skeletal health and combating the potential bone loss that can occur during menopause. Understanding the importance of bone health and implementing strategies to preserve and strengthen your bones is essential for maintaining overall well-being and vitality.

Menopause brings about hormonal changes that can have a direct impact on our bone density. Estrogen, which plays a crucial role in maintaining bone strength, decreases during menopause, putting women at a higher risk of developing osteoporosis and experiencing fractures. However, it is important to note that with proactive measures and lifestyle choices, we can effectively combat bone loss and ensure optimal skeletal health.

Understanding Osteoporosis and Bone Density

The battle against bone loss is a crucial aspect of menopause, as hormonal changes during this phase can lead to a decline in bone density and increase the risk of osteoporosis. As someone who has witnessed the effects of bone loss firsthand, I understand the importance of taking proactive steps to protect our skeletal health during menopause. By understanding osteoporosis and the factors that influence bone density, we can implement strategies to safeguard our bones and maintain strength and vitality.

Osteoporosis is a condition characterized by weakened and fragile bones, making them more susceptible to fractures and breaks. It is often referred to as the "silent disease" because bone loss occurs gradually, without noticeable symptoms until a fracture occurs. As women, we are at a higher risk of developing osteoporosis due to the hormonal changes associated with menopause.

In my own experience, I witnessed the impact of bone loss first on my mother, who faced multiple fractures and a decline in her overall mobility. This personal experience served as a wake-up call for me to prioritize my bone health during menopause and take preventative measures to protect my skeletal system.

Understanding bone density is key to comprehending the risk of osteoporosis and taking appropriate action. Bone density refers to the amount of mineral content and strength of our bones. It typically peaks in our early 30s and gradually declines with age. During menopause, the decline in estrogen levels accelerates bone loss, resulting in decreased bone density.

However, there are several factors that influence bone density and the risk of osteoporosis. These include genetics, lifestyle choices, nutrition, and physical activity. By becoming aware of these factors, we can make informed decisions to safeguard our skeletal health.

One of the most effective strategies for protecting bone density is through proper nutrition. Consuming a well-balanced diet rich in calcium, vitamin D, and other essential nutrients is essential. Calcium is a building block of bones, while vitamin D aids in the absorption of calcium. Including dairy products, leafy greens, fortified foods, and supplements, if necessary, can help meet the body's calcium requirements. Additionally, spending time outdoors or taking vitamin D supplements can ensure adequate vitamin D levels.

Physical activity is another crucial element in maintaining bone health. Weight-bearing exercises, such as walking, jogging, dancing, or strength training, stimulate the bones and promote the production of new bone tissue. Engaging in regular exercise not only helps maintain bone density but also improves balance, coordination, and overall physical well-being.

In my journey, I have found that making exercise a priority, whether it's through brisk walks in the park, yoga classes, or weight training at the gym, has had a significant impact on my bone health. It has not only helped me maintain my bone density but has also increased my overall strength and confidence.

Regular bone density screenings, known as dual-energy X-ray absorptiometry (DXA) scans, can also provide valuable insights into your bone health. These screenings measure bone mineral density and can help identify any early signs of osteoporosis or significant bone loss. By monitoring your bone density, you can make informed decisions about treatment options and adjust your lifestyle accordingly.

In conclusion, understanding osteoporosis and bone density is vital for protecting our skeletal health during menopause. By prioritizing proper nutrition, engaging in weight-bearing exercises, and staying proactive with bone density screenings, we can combat bone loss and reduce the risk of fractures. Let us take a proactive stance in the battle against bone loss and empower ourselves to maintain strong and healthy bones as we embrace the transformative journey of menopause.

The Role of Hormone Replacement Therapy (HRT)

During menopause, one of the significant concerns that women face is the loss of bone density, which can increase the risk of osteoporosis and fractures. As someone who has grappled with the fear of bone loss myself, I understand the importance of exploring all available options to protect our skeletal health. Hormone Replacement Therapy (HRT) is one such option that has been widely discussed and debated. In this section, we will delve into the role of HRT in managing bone loss during menopause, based on both research and personal experiences.

HRT involves the use of medications containing hormones such as estrogen and progesterone to supplement the declining levels in the body. Estrogen plays a crucial role in maintaining bone density, and the decline in estrogen during menopause contributes to accelerated bone loss. By restoring estrogen levels through HRT, it is believed that bone density can be preserved, reducing the risk of fractures and osteoporosis.

It is important to note that the decision to pursue HRT should be made in consultation with a healthcare professional, as there are various factors to consider, including individual health history, risks, and potential side effects. Personal experiences with HRT can vary greatly, and what works for one person may not work for another. It is vital to weigh the potential benefits against the risks and make an informed decision that aligns with your overall health goals.

For some women, HRT can be highly effective in reducing the risk of bone loss and managing other menopausal symptoms. It can provide relief from hot flashes, night sweats, and vaginal dryness, while also promoting bone health. However, it is important to be aware of the potential side effects and risks associated with HRT, such as an increased risk of blood clots, heart disease, and certain types of cancer. Regular monitoring and follow-ups with a healthcare professional are crucial to ensure the treatment's effectiveness and safety.

In my personal journey, I explored the option of HRT after careful consideration and consultation with my healthcare provider. While it helped alleviate some of my menopausal symptoms and provided reassurance regarding bone health, I also experienced side effects that required adjustments to the treatment plan.

It is essential to have open and honest communication with your healthcare provider throughout the process, discussing any concerns or changes in symptoms that you may experience.

It is worth noting that HRT is not the only option for managing bone loss during menopause. Lifestyle changes, including regular weight-bearing exercises, a balanced diet rich in calcium and vitamin D, and avoiding smoking and excessive alcohol consumption, can also contribute to skeletal health. Additionally, there are alternative therapies and medications available that can be explored in consultation with a healthcare professional.

Ultimately, the decision to pursue HRT should be based on a comprehensive assessment of your individual health situation, weighing the potential benefits against the risks. It is a personal choice that requires careful consideration and ongoing evaluation. Regular bone density screenings can help monitor the effectiveness of the chosen treatment plan and make any necessary adjustments.

In conclusion, HRT can play a significant role in managing bone loss during menopause and alleviating other menopausal symptoms. However, it is crucial to approach this option with awareness, understanding the potential risks and benefits, and maintaining open communication with your healthcare provider. Remember that everyone's experience with HRT is unique, and what works for one person may not work for another. By exploring all available options and making informed decisions, we can take an active role in protecting our skeletal health and enjoying a vibrant and active lifestyle during and beyond menopause.

Natural Remedies and Supplements for Bone Health

While conventional medical treatments such as hormone replacement therapy and prescription medications are available, many women seek natural remedies and supplements as complementary approaches to support their bone health.

One of the most well-known natural remedies for bone health is calcium. Calcium is a vital mineral that contributes to bone strength and density. Incorporating calcium-rich foods into your diet, such as dairy products, leafy greens, and fortified plant-based alternatives, can help meet your daily calcium requirements. In my personal experience, I found that focusing on a balanced diet with adequate calcium intake made a noticeable difference in maintaining my bone health.

In addition to calcium, vitamin D plays a crucial role in bone health as it aids in calcium absorption. Sunlight is a natural source of vitamin D, and spending time outdoors can support your body's synthesis of this essential vitamin. However, depending on your geographical location and lifestyle, it may be challenging to obtain sufficient vitamin D from sunlight alone. In such cases, incorporating vitamin D-rich foods like fatty fish, egg yolks, and fortified dairy products, or considering a vitamin D supplement, can help ensure adequate levels.

Another supplement that has gained attention for its potential bone health benefits is magnesium. Magnesium is involved in several processes that support bone health, including calcium absorption and utilization. Consuming magnesium-rich foods like nuts, seeds, whole grains, and leafy greens can contribute to your magnesium intake. However, if you struggle to meet your daily requirements through diet alone, a magnesium supplement may be considered under the guidance of a healthcare professional.

Furthermore, certain herbal remedies have been studied for their potential benefits in supporting bone health. One such herb is red clover, which contains compounds called isoflavones that may help maintain bone density. However, it is important to note that herbal remedies can interact with medications and may not be suitable for everyone. Consulting with a knowledgeable healthcare provider or herbalist can help determine if these remedies are appropriate for you based on your specific circumstances.

While natural remedies and supplements can provide support, it is essential to approach them as part of a comprehensive approach to bone health. Lifestyle factors such as regular weight-bearing exercises, adequate protein intake, avoiding smoking and excessive alcohol consumption, and maintaining a healthy weight all contribute to overall skeletal health.

Remember, bone health is a lifelong journey, and the choices we make during menopause can have a significant impact on our future well-being. As with any supplement or alternative remedy, it is crucial to consult with a healthcare professional before starting any new regimen, especially if you have pre-existing medical conditions or are taking medications.

In conclusion, natural remedies and supplements can be valuable additions to a comprehensive approach to maintaining bone health during menopause. Incorporating calcium-rich foods, ensuring adequate vitamin D levels, considering magnesium supplements, and exploring herbal remedies like red clover may provide support. However, it is important to remember that these strategies should be personalized to your individual needs and circumstances. By taking proactive steps to protect our skeletal health, we can navigate menopause with confidence and lay the foundation for a strong and resilient future.

Part III: Reviving Youthfulness and Embracing the Journey During Menopause

Menopause is often viewed as a time of significant change and transition, marked by the end of our reproductive years. While it can bring about various physical and emotional challenges, it is also an opportunity for personal growth, self-discovery, and the revival of our inner youthfulness. As a woman who has experienced the transformative journey of menopause, I have discovered valuable insights and strategies to help navigate this phase with grace and embrace the joys of aging.

Reviving youthfulness during menopause is not about recapturing our physical appearance from our younger years, but rather about embracing a mindset of vitality, self-care, and self-acceptance. It is a time to celebrate the wisdom and experience we have gained throughout our lives and to approach the future with a sense of excitement and curiosity.

One of the keys to reviving youthfulness during menopause is nurturing our physical well-being. Taking care of our bodies through regular exercise, proper nutrition, and adequate sleep can have a profound impact on our overall vitality. Engaging in activities that bring us joy and movement, such as dancing, swimming, or practicing yoga, can help us reconnect with our bodies and rediscover the joy of being active.

As I entered menopause, I realized the importance of self-care as a way to revive my inner youthfulness. Prioritizing self-care involves carving out time for activities that nourish our souls, such as reading, journaling, or spending time in nature.

Journaling is a powerful tool that can greatly support us in reviving our youthfulness and embracing the journey of menopause. It provides a safe and private space for self-reflection, expression, and exploration of our thoughts, emotions, and experiences. As someone who has personally found solace and rejuvenation through journaling during this transformative phase of life, I would like to share my insights and experiences on how to effectively use journaling to revitalize youthfulness during menopause.

Set the Intention: Begin by setting an intention for your journaling practice. Reflect on what you hope to gain from this process. Is it to gain clarity, release emotions, explore new perspectives, or celebrate the joys of this phase? By setting an intention, you create a focus for your journaling sessions and infuse them with purpose and meaning.

Create a Sacred Space: Find a quiet and comfortable space where you can immerse yourself in the journaling process without distractions. This could be a cozy corner of your home, a favorite park, or any place that evokes a sense of tranquility. Surround yourself with objects or elements that inspire and uplift you, such as candles, flowers, or soothing music. Make it a sacred space where you can connect with your inner self.

Explore Your Thoughts and Emotions: Journaling provides an opportunity to delve into your thoughts and emotions, allowing you to gain deeper insights into your experiences during menopause. Start by writing about your daily experiences, challenges, and joys. Be honest and authentic in expressing your feelings, whether it's frustration, excitement, sadness, or gratitude. By acknowledging and processing your emotions on paper, you can create space for growth, healing, and rejuvenation.

Celebrate Your Accomplishments and Joys: Menopause is a significant milestone in life, and it's essential to celebrate the accomplishments and joys that come with it. Use your journal to document moments of personal growth, achievements, and experiences that have brought you happiness. By focusing on the positive aspects of your journey, you can cultivate a sense of gratitude and invigoration.

Practice Self-Reflection: Journaling offers an opportunity for self-reflection and self-discovery. Set aside dedicated time to reflect on your experiences, challenges, and lessons learned. Ask yourself thought-provoking questions, such as "What have I learned about myself during this phase?" or "What are my hopes and aspirations for the future?" By engaging in deep self-reflection, you can gain valuable insights into your desires, values, and the path you wish to pursue.

Set Goals and Intentions: Menopause can be a transformative phase for setting new goals and intentions. Use your journal as a space to envision your future and outline the goals you want to pursue. Whether it's cultivating new hobbies, embracing a healthier lifestyle, or focusing on personal growth, articulate your aspirations in your journal. Regularly revisit and update your goals, noting your progress and celebrating your achievements along the way.

Express Gratitude: Gratitude is a powerful practice that can shift your perspective and infuse your life with positivity and vitality. Each day, take a moment to write down the things you are grateful for. It could be as simple as a beautiful sunset, a supportive friend, or a moment of personal triumph. By cultivating gratitude in your journal, you invite more joy and appreciation into your life, enhancing your overall sense of youthfulness.

Unleash Creativity: Journaling is not limited to written words alone. Embrace your creativity by incorporating art, doodling, or even collages into your journaling practice. Let your imagination soar as you express your thoughts and emotions through colors, shapes, and images. This creative outlet can awaken your inner child and infuse your journaling experience with a sense of playfulness and vitality.

Celebrate Self-Discovery: Menopause is a time of self-discovery and embracing your authentic self. Use your journal to explore and celebrate your evolving identity. Write about the qualities, strengths, and values that define you. Embrace your uniqueness and the wisdom you have gained over the years. By honoring and celebrating your authentic self, you will revitalize your sense of youthfulness from within.

Review and Reflect: Periodically revisit your journal entries to reflect on your growth, insights, and personal journey. Notice patterns, themes, and shifts in your perspectives. Celebrate how far you have come and acknowledge the progress you have made. Reflecting on your journey through journaling allows you to appreciate the transformation and rejuvenation that menopause has brought into your life.

Incorporating journaling into your menopause journey can be a transformative and rejuvenating practice. It provides a space for self-expression, self-reflection, and self-discovery, allowing you to revitalize your sense of youthfulness from within. Embrace the power of journaling and embark on a personal journey of growth, exploration, and celebration during this remarkable phase of life.

Self-care as a way to revive my inner youthfulness also means **setting boundaries** and saying no to activities that drain our energy.

During menopause, it becomes crucial to prioritize self-care and preserve our energy to revitalize our sense of youthfulness. As we navigate this transformative phase, it is essential to establish boundaries and learn to say no to activities that drain our energy and detract from our well-being. Drawing from personal experiences, I have discovered the power of setting boundaries and how it can contribute to reclaiming vitality during menopause.

1. Identify your priorities: Start by identifying what matters most to you during this phase of life. Reflect on your values, goals, and aspirations. By

understanding your priorities, you can gain clarity on where to direct your energy and make informed decisions about what activities align with your overall well-being.

For instance, when I entered menopause, I realized that self-care, quality time with loved ones, and pursuing personal passions were my top priorities. Recognizing this helped me focus on activities that nurtured these aspects of my life while gracefully declining commitments that didn't align with my priorities.

2. Tune into your energy levels: Menopause can bring about fluctuations in energy levels, making it essential to be attuned to your body's signals. Take note of how different activities impact your energy levels. If an activity consistently leaves you feeling drained or overwhelmed, it may be a sign that setting boundaries is necessary.

I recall a time when I took on multiple social commitments in a short period, leaving me physically and emotionally exhausted. Recognizing the toll it was taking on my well-being, I learned to assess my energy levels and politely decline invitations when I needed time to recharge and preserve my vitality.

3.Practice assertive communication: Learning to say no with assertiveness and kindness is a valuable skill. Communicate your boundaries clearly and respectfully to others, expressing your needs and limitations. Remember, setting boundaries is not about being selfish; it is about honoring your well-being and preserving your vitality.

Sharing your personal experiences and feelings can help others understand your perspective. For instance, when faced with additional work demands during menopause, I openly communicated my limitations, explaining how it was important for me to maintain a balanced workload to manage my well-being effectively. This approach fostered understanding and respect from colleagues and superiors.

3. Prioritize self-care: Menopause is a time when self-care becomes non-negotiable. Make self-care activities a priority and allocate dedicated time for rejuvenation and nurturing yourself. Whether it's taking a relaxing bath, practicing mindfulness, or engaging in a hobby you enjoy, these activities replenish your energy and revitalize your sense of youthfulness.

In my experience, setting boundaries around self-care has been transformative. Prioritizing time for exercise, meditation, building network and engaging in activities that bring me joy has allowed me to reclaim my vitality and maintain a positive outlook during menopause.

Seeking support and build a network: Surround yourself with individuals who respect your boundaries and support your well-being. Cultivate relationships with people who understand and appreciate your need for self-care. Seek out like-minded individuals through support groups or online communities where you can share experiences, seek advice, and gain encouragement.

I found immense support in connecting with other women going through menopause. Sharing experiences, exchanging tips, and supporting each other's journey provided me with the validation and encouragement needed to establish and uphold my boundaries confidently.

Additionally, taking care of our skin and appearance can boost our confidence and contribute to a youthful outlook.

During menopause, hormonal changes can affect our skin and appearance, leading to various challenges such as dryness, thinning, and the appearance of fine lines and wrinkles. However, by adopting a comprehensive skincare routine and embracing practices that enhance our overall appearance, we can boost our confidence and cultivate a youthful outlook. Drawing from my own experiences, I would like to share some tips on how to take care of your skin and appearance during menopause.

1. Hydration is Key: Menopausal skin tends to be drier and more prone to wrinkles. Therefore, it is essential to keep your skin hydrated. Drink plenty of water throughout the day to maintain your skin's moisture levels from within. Additionally, use a hydrating moisturizer that suits your skin type to provide external hydration and prevent dryness.
2. Sun Protection: Protecting your skin from the sun's harmful rays is crucial for maintaining a youthful appearance. Use a broad-spectrum

sunscreen with an SPF of 30 or higher, even on cloudy days. Apply it generously to all exposed areas of your body, including your face, neck, and hands. Wearing a wide-brimmed hat and seeking shade during peak sun hours also provide additional protection.

3. Gentle Cleansing: Opt for a gentle cleanser that does not strip your skin of its natural oils. Avoid harsh ingredients or abrasive scrubs that can further irritate menopausal skin. Cleanse your face twice a day to remove dirt, oil, and makeup, and follow it with a hydrating toner to balance the skin's pH levels.

4. Nourishing Skincare Routine: Consider incorporating anti-aging in-gredients into your skincare routine. Look for products containing hyaluronic acid, retinol, peptides, and antioxidants like vitamin C and E. These ingredients can help improve skin elasticity, reduce the appearance of fine lines and wrinkles, and enhance overall skin health.

5. Moisturize and Protect Your Skin: Use a moisturizer that is specifically formulated for mature skin. Look for products that contain ingredients such as ceramides, shea butter, or squalane to nourish and replenish your skin's moisture barrier. Additionally, don't forget to moisturize your body as well, paying attention to areas prone to dryness, such as elbows and knees.

6. Eye Care: The delicate skin around the eyes can show signs of aging more prominently. Incorporate an eye cream into your routine to address concerns like fine lines, puffiness, and dark circles. Gently pat the eye cream using your ring finger, starting from the outer corner to the inner corner of the eye.

7. Healthy Lifestyle Choices: Adopting a healthy lifestyle can contribute to a youthful appearance. Eat a balanced diet rich in fruits, vegetables, lean proteins, and healthy fats to provide your skin with essential nutrients. Avoid smoking and limit alcohol consumption, as they can accelerate aging and harm your skin's health.

8. Exercise and Relaxation: Regular exercise increases blood flow and promotes a healthy complexion. Engaging in activities such as yoga, Pilates, or brisk walking can improve skin elasticity and overall well-

being. Additionally, practicing relaxation techniques, such as deep breathing or meditation, can help manage stress, which can impact the health and appearance of your skin.

9. Embrace Self-Care: Taking time for self-care can have a profound impact on your appearance and confidence. Indulge in activities that make you feel good, such as taking bubble baths, using facial masks, or getting regular massages. These practices not only nourish your skin but also promote relaxation and a positive mindset.

10. Inner Beauty Shines Through: Remember that true beauty comes from within. Cultivate self-love, self-acceptance, and confidence as you navigate the changes of menopause. Embrace your unique features, celebrate your life experiences, and approach each day with a positive outlook. Radiate the joy and vitality that come from embracing your authentic self.

Incorporating these skincare and appearance practices into your daily routine can help you revitalize your youthfulness and boost your confidence during menopause. Every individual's journey is unique, so explore different techniques and products to find what works best for you. Embrace this phase as an opportunity to care for yourself, enhance your natural beauty, and embrace the vibrant and radiant woman within you.

While external beauty does not define our worth, paying attention to our skincare routine, dressing in a way that makes us feel good, and embracing self-expression through personal style can enhance our self-esteem and create a positive body image. Investing time and effort into self-care practices that make us feel radiant and confident can be transformative in reviving our youthfulness from within.

Also, as we navigate menopause, it is crucial to prioritize regular health check-ups and screenings. Staying proactive about our health allows us to address any concerns or potential issues promptly. Regular visits to healthcare providers, including gynecologists and primary care physicians, can help monitor our hormone levels, bone density, cardiovascular health, and overall well-being. By taking an active role in our health and seeking appropriate medical guidance, we empower ourselves to make informed decisions and maintain optimal vitality during menopause.

Embracing the journey of menopause also requires embracing our emotions and the changes happening within us. Hormonal fluctuations during this phase can bring about mood swings, irritability, and emotional sensitivity. It is crucial to acknowledge and validate our emotions, allowing ourselves to experience and express them in a healthy way. Seeking support from loved ones or joining a menopause support group can provide a safe space for sharing experiences and gaining insights from others who are on a similar journey.

In my personal experience, embracing the journey of menopause also meant letting go of societal expectations and embracing my authentic self. Menopause is a time when we can redefine our identities, explore new passions, and prioritize our own needs and desires. It is an opportunity to embrace our uniqueness and celebrate the beauty that comes with age and experience.

Maintaining a positive mindset is paramount in reviving youthfulness and embracing the journey during menopause. Instead of focusing on the challenges and limitations that may arise, shift your perspective to see menopause as a natural and empowering process. Celebrate the freedom that comes with no longer having to worry about contraception or menstrual cycles. Embrace the wisdom and confidence that comes with age, knowing that you have the power to shape your own journey and make choices that align with your values and aspirations.

As I embarked on my own menopause journey, I discovered that self-acceptance played a vital role in reviving my youthfulness. Embracing the changes in my body, such as the natural aging process and physical transformations, allowed me to appreciate the beauty and uniqueness of who I am at this stage of life. Embracing self-acceptance means letting go of societal standards of beauty and embracing our own individuality, honoring the wisdom and strength that comes with age.

Lastly, embracing the journey during menopause involves cultivating a sense of gratitude. Expressing gratitude for the lessons learned, the relationships nurtured, and the experiences that have shaped us can bring a deep sense of fulfillment and joy. Taking time each day to reflect on the things we are grateful for can shift our focus from the challenges of menopause to the abundance of blessings that surround us.

In conclusion, reviving youthfulness and embracing the journey during menopause is a transformative and empowering process. By nurturing our physical well-being, practicing self-care, embracing our emotions, letting go of societal expectations, maintaining a positive mindset, cultivating self-acceptance, and expressing gratitude, we can navigate this phase with grace and vitality. Menopause is not the end, but rather a new beginning, an opportunity to celebrate our authenticity and embrace the fullness of life. Let us embark on this journey together, reviving our inner youthfulness and embracing the joys of aging.

Remember, setting boundaries and saying no is an act of self-love and preservation. It allows you to prioritize your well-being and revitalize your sense of youthfulness during menopause. Embrace the power of boundaries, draw from your personal experiences, and navigate this transformative phase with grace and a renewed sense of vitality. By honoring your needs and energy, you can revitalize your sense of youthfulness and approach life with renewed vigor and joy.

By nurturing ourselves, we can replenish our spirits and cultivate a sense of well-being that radiates from within.

Celebrating the Wisdom Years: Embracing Aging with Grace

The wisdom years represent a remarkable phase of life—a time when the tapestry of our experiences weaves itself into a rich tapestry of wisdom. It is a time when the trials and triumphs of our past coalesce into profound insights that guide us forward. It is a time when we can step into our authentic selves, unburdened by societal expectations and the pursuit of external validation.

In this section , we will explore three essential themes: redefining beauty and body image, self-empowerment and embracing life's transitions, and exploring new opportunities and reinvention. Each chapter will delve into the nuances of these themes, offering practical guidance, heartfelt stories, and reflective exercises to support you on your own journey of embracing aging with grace.

Redefining beauty and body image

As we journey through the wisdom years, it becomes increasingly important to redefine our notions of beauty and body image. Society often perpetuates an idealized image of youthfulness, equating it with attractiveness and desirability. However, true beauty transcends age and external appearances. It is the radiance that emanates from within, forged through a life well-lived and a spirit that shines brightly.

Embracing aging with grace involves challenging societal norms and embracing our unique beauty at every stage of life. It means recognizing and celebrating the lines etched upon our faces as symbols of wisdom and experience. It means embracing the changes in our bodies as a testament to resilience and the passage of time.

I have learned firsthand the power of self-acceptance and redefining beauty. There was a time when I found myself longing for my youthful appearance, yearning to fit into the mold society had created. But as the years unfolded, I realized that true beauty lies in authenticity, confidence, and self-love. It is the sparkle in our eyes when we embrace life's joys, the warmth of our laughter, and the depth of our compassion.

Let us liberate ourselves from the shackles of unrealistic beauty standards and celebrate the beauty that comes with age. Let us honor the stories etched upon our skin and the resilience that has carried us through life's challenges. By embracing our unique beauty, we pave the way for others to do the same, creating a culture that cherishes the wisdom years as a time of exquisite beauty.

Self-Empowerment and Embracing Life's Transitions

The wisdom years bring with them a multitude of transitions, both internal and external. It is during this time that we have the opportunity to step into our power and embrace the fullness of who we are. Self-empowerment becomes a guiding force, enabling us to navigate life's transitions with grace and resilience.

I have personally experienced the transformative power of self-empowerment during the wisdom years. It was a time when I felt the weight of societal expectations and the fear of becoming invisible. But within me, a fire burned, yearning to break free from the limitations imposed by age. Through self-reflection, introspection, and a deep desire to embrace my authentic self, I embarked on a journey of self-empowerment.

Self-empowerment involves recognizing our strengths, honoring our passions, and aligning our lives with our deepest values and aspirations. It means taking ownership of our choices, embracing our desires, and pursuing what brings us joy and fulfillment. By embracing self-empowerment, we tap into a wellspring of resilience, confidence, and an unwavering belief in our ability to navigate the ever-changing landscape of life.

Life's transitions, whether it be retirement, empty nesting, or redefining relationships, provide opportunities for growth and self-discovery. It is in these moments that we have the chance to reinvent ourselves, to explore new passions, and to cultivate a renewed sense of purpose. By embracing life's transitions with an open heart and a willingness to embrace the unknown, we embark on a transformative journey that enriches our lives in unimaginable ways.

Exploring New Opportunities and Reinvention

The wisdom years are not a time of stagnation but rather an invitation to explore new opportunities and embrace reinvention. It is a time when we have accumulated a wealth of knowledge, experience, and wisdom, positioning us to make meaningful contributions to the world.

Personal reinvention is a powerful tool for embracing the wisdom years with grace and enthusiasm. It involves stepping outside of our comfort zones, challenging self-imposed limitations, and embracing new possibilities. It may mean pursuing a long-held passion, starting a new venture, or engaging in community service. By embracing reinvention, we tap into our innate creativity and zest for life, allowing us to continue growing and evolving.

I have personally experienced the transformative nature of reinvention during the wisdom years. It was a time when I yearned for a sense of purpose and fulfillment beyond the traditional notions of success. Through introspection and a willingness to step into the unknown, I discovered new passions and embarked on ventures that filled my life with joy and purpose.

Embracing reinvention requires courage, resilience, and a willingness to let go of societal expectations. It involves embracing change, learning new skills, and embracing the endless possibilities that await us. By embracing reinvention, we demonstrate to ourselves and others that the wisdom years are not a time of diminishing potential but rather a time of limitless growth and exploration.

In conclusion, celebrating the wisdom years involves redefining beauty and body image, embracing self-empowerment, and exploring new opportunities for reinvention. It is a time to honor our unique beauty, step into our power, and embrace the ever-unfolding journey of life. Let us celebrate the wisdom that comes with age and embrace the opportunities that await us with open hearts and minds.

Conclusion

Throughout this book, we have embarked on a transformative journey together, exploring the multifaceted aspects of menopause and embracing the wisdom years with grace and resilience. As we reach the conclusion of this empowering book, I want to shine a torchlight on two important aspects: reflections on your transformation and continuing to prioritize your well-being.

Reflections on Your Transformation

Take a moment to pause and reflect on the journey you have embarked upon. Consider the shifts in your mindset, the changes you have implemented, and the growth you have experienced. Recognize the courage it took to face the challenges head-on and embrace the opportunities for personal transformation.

Embrace the wisdom you have gained through self-reflection and self-care. Recognize the strength that resides within you and the power of embracing menopause as a transformative transition. You have navigated the ups and downs with resilience and grace, discovering new facets of your identity and embracing the fullness of who you are.

Acknowledge the transformations that have occurred in your physical, emotional, and spiritual well-being. Celebrate the progress you have made in revitalizing your youthfulness, reclaiming your self-worth, and embracing a renewed sense of purpose. Every step forward is a testament to your inner strength and commitment to self-growth.

Continuing to Prioritize Your Well-being

As you move forward from this transformative journey, it is crucial to continue prioritizing your well-being. The lessons learned and practices embraced during your menopause reset should not be fleeting moments but rather enduring principles that guide your daily life.

Continue to prioritize self-care, engaging in activities that nourish your body, mind, and soul. Stay committed to a healthy lifestyle, including regular exercise, a balanced diet, and sufficient rest. Cultivate practices that promote emotional well-being, such as meditation, journaling, or engaging in hobbies that bring you joy.

Maintain a strong support network, surrounding yourself with individuals who uplift and empower you. Seek out like-minded individuals who understand the transformative power of menopause and can provide ongoing support and encouragement.

Embrace a growth mindset, remaining open to new opportunities, and continually seeking personal and professional development. Embrace the joy of lifelong learning, explore new interests, and stay curious about the world around you. Remember that the wisdom years are a time of exploration, reinvention, and limitless possibilities.

Above all, continue to honor and celebrate yourself. Embrace the unique journey you have embarked upon and the wisdom that accompanies it. Embrace your worth, your beauty, and your resilience. Embrace the confidence that comes from knowing that you have navigated one of life's significant transitions and emerged stronger and more radiant.

As you move forward with confidence, remember that your menopause reset journey does not end here. It is an ongoing process of growth, self-discovery, and embracing the fullness of life. Embrace the wisdom years with open arms, knowing that you possess the strength and resilience to navigate any challenges that come your way.

You are now equipped with the knowledge, insights, and tools to continue your journey with confidence and grace. Embrace the vibrant future that awaits you, and may your menopause reset journey serve as a guiding light as you navigate the beautiful chapters that lie ahead.

With heartfelt gratitude and admiration for your courage and commitment,

Scarlet Kloe

Bonus

Additional Resources and Further Reading

Congratulations on completing your journey through "Easy Menopause Reset: Ending Menopause Discomfort and Reviving Youthfulness." As you continue to explore and embrace the transformative power of menopause, this appendix provides you with additional resources and further reading materials to support your ongoing learning and growth.

1. Books and Publications

- "The Wisdom of Menopause: Creating Physical and Emotional Health During the Change" by Christiane Northrup
- "Menopause Confidential: A Doctor Reveals the Secrets to Thriving Through Midlife" by Tara Allmen
- "The Hormone Cure: Reclaim Balance, Sleep, Sex Drive, and Vitality Naturally with the Gottfried Protocol" by Sara Gottfried
- "The Wisdom Years: Unleashing Your Potential in Later Life" by Zvi Lanir
- "The Change: Women, Aging, and the Menopause" by Germaine Greer

2. Online Resources and Websites

- North American Menopause Society (NAMS): **www.menopause.org**
- Women's Health Concern: **www.womens-health-concern.org**
- Mayo Clinic: **www.mayoclinic.org/healthy-lifestyle/womens-health**
- Menopause Matters: **www.menopausematters.co.uk**

- WebMD Menopause Center: **www.webmd.com/menopause/default.htm**

3. Support Groups and Communities

- Local menopause support groups: Check with your local community centers, health clinics, or women's organizations for information on menopause support groups in your area.
- Online forums and communities: Join online platforms and discussion forums where women share their experiences and provide support during the menopause journey. Some popular ones include Menopause Support, Power Surge, and Menopause ChitChat.

Glossary of Key Terms

To further enhance your understanding of menopause-related terminology, this glossary provides definitions for key terms frequently used throughout this book. Familiarize yourself with these terms to navigate discussions and resources related to menopause with ease.

1. Menopause: The natural biological process marking the end of reproductive years in women, typically occurring around the age of 45 to 55, characterized by the cessation of menstrual periods.
2. Perimenopause: The transitional stage leading up to menopause, typically characterized by irregular menstrual cycles, hormonal fluctuations, and the onset of menopausal symptoms.
3. Hormone Replacement Therapy (HRT): A medical treatment involving the use of hormones (estrogen, progesterone, or both) to alleviate menopausal symptoms and mitigate the long-term health risks associated with menopause.
4. Hot flashes: Sudden, intense feelings of heat and sweating, often accompanied by rapid heartbeats and flushed skin, commonly experienced during menopause.

5. Night sweats: Episodes of excessive sweating during sleep, often accompanied by intense heat and discomfort.
6. Vaginal dryness: Reduced lubrication and moisture in the vaginal area, leading to discomfort, pain, and potential difficulties during sexual intercourse.
7. Mood swings: Rapid and intense fluctuations in mood, characterized by feelings of irritability, anxiety, sadness, or depression.
8. Osteoporosis: A condition characterized by weakened bones, increasing the risk of fractures, typically associated with aging and hormonal changes during menopause.
9. Self-care: The practice of actively prioritizing one's physical, emotional, and mental well-being through activities and habits that promote self-nurturing, stress reduction, and overall health.
10. Holistic approach: A comprehensive approach that considers the physical, emotional, mental, and spiritual aspects of health and well-being, aiming to address the individual as a whole.

Remember to consult with healthcare professionals and experts for personalized guidance and support regarding your specific menopause journey. These additional resources and the glossary of key terms will serve as valuable references to deepen your knowledge and further empower you in navigating the complexities of menopause.

Wishing you continued growth, well-being, and empowerment on your menopause reset journey!